Von Willebrand Disease:
Fast Focus Study Guide

JT Thomas, MD

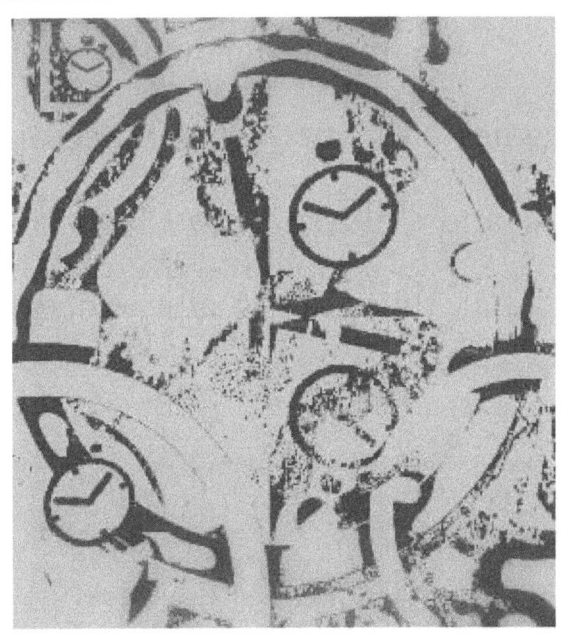

Acknowledgements

I dedicate this book to my beautiful
wife and children, who I love more
than all the water in all the oceans
and all the seas.

CONTENTS

- This book is written to help the reader further understand von Willebrand Disease.

- This book is written in a simple and easy to read format designed for medical students, residents and physicians who are preparing for boards.

- This book simplifies a complicated medical issue so you will remember the important details.

- You will not get caught up in the minutia. Just the facts are found in this book.

- This Fast Focus Study Guide will provide you with a practical review of the key information you need to know.

- Buy this book now if you want this quick and concise information

Von Willebrand disease is characterized by insufficient or ineffective von Willebrand factor leading to impaired platelet adhesion and deficient factor VIII levels.

Von Willebrand factor is a multimeric glycoprotein that acts as a bridging molecule at sites of vascular injury for normal platelet adhesion and promotes platelet aggregation. This protein also functions as a carrier that stabilized factor VIII in circulation.

Von Willebrand disease (vWD) is the most common autosomally inherited bleeding disorder.

VWD causes symptoms in about in 1 in 1000

people.

VWD is more common and usually milder than hemophilia.

VWD is characterized by clinical symptoms including excessive mucocutaneous bleeding.

Unlike diseases like sickle cell or thalassemia, VWD has no geographical or ethnic characteristics.

Males and females inherit the mutant von Willebrand factor alleles with equal frequency however females are more commonly diagnosed likely related to factors exclusive to females such as excessive menstrual bleeding.

There are three forms of vWD: inherited, acquired, and pseudo or platelet type.

Von Willebrand protein is produced by the endothelium and in megakaryocytes. It is found in arterioles. It is not found in veins, capillaries, or large arteries.

Characteristic laboratory parameters can help identify people with von Willebrand disease.

The PT is normal in patients with von Willebrand's disease.

Individuals with VWD will also have normal platelet counts, thrombin time, and fibrinogen levels.

The von Willebrand factor activity is usually assessed based on measurement of the ristocetin cofactor (von Willebrand factor:RCo).

A prolonged aPTT is characteristic of VWD, however a normal aPTT does not exclude this diagnosis.

It is important to remember that both hemophilia A and vWD are associated with decreased levels of factor VIII.

Patients with a prolonged aPTT as well as patients who have symptoms or family history that are suspicious for VWD should be tested for von Willebrand factor antigen (von Willebrand factor:Ag), ristocetin cofactor activity (von Willebrand factor:RCo), and factor VIII activity.

The thrombin time is not affected by von Willebrand's disease.

Mixing studies are characterized by a prolonged aPTT that normalizes immediately after mixing with normal plasma, and does not reverse after incubation is consistent with VWD.

A prolonged aPTT that remains prolonged after mixing with normal plasma or an aPTT that normalizes immediately after mixing with normal plasma but prolongs after incubation is not characteristic of VWD.

VWD can rarely be acquired, but most often is inherited in an autosomal fashion.

The gene for von Willebrand factor is located on the short arm of chromosome 12.

Since type 1 and 2 are autosomal dominant, these patients will have only one parent with a vWD.

VWD type 3 is autosomal recessive and therefore both parents have to contribute the genetic mutation.

Hemophilia A is sometimes part of the differential diagnosis for vWD. It is helpful to remember that hemophilia is an X linked recessive disease (only males).

Hereditary hemorrhagic telangiectasia can be associated with increased incidence of vWD.

DDAVP is usually only effective in Von Willebrand Disease patients with type 1 Von Willebrand Disease

Type 1 VWD is characterized by a quantitative deficiency of von Willebrand factor. Type 1 vWD accounts for 65% to 75% of VWD.

Type 1 vWD can have von Willebrand factor levels can vary from person to person and range from 5% to 40% depending on the molecular pathogenesis.

Mucocutaneous bleeding is generally mild in type 1 vWD.

Some patients with type 1 vWD will have essential no symptoms and most patients will have a nearly normal life with only mild symptoms if present.

Some people with Type I vWD can have significant bleeding with trauma, surgery, or with tooth extraction.

Many patients with type 1 vWD are never diagnosed due to the asymptomatic or mild presentation and are unaware they have vWD.

In type 1 vWD the von Willebrand factor variants are most often missense substitutions affecting von Willebrand factor, storage, secretion, trafficking, and clearance.

During pregnancy the level of von Willebrand factor increases in most women with types 1 and 2 vWD and labor and delivery usually not associated with excessive bleeding.

Type 2 von Willebrand type 2 disease is characterized by the expression of dysfunctional von Willebrand factor and occurs in 20% to 35% of patients.

The von Willebrand factor levels in type 2 are usually normal but they do not function correctly.

Type 2 vWD divided into subtypes: 2A, 2B, 2M, and 2N. Each subtype is characterized by a different gene mutation.

Type 2 vWD is usually are inherited in a dominant fashion with the exception of type IIN which is inherited in an autosomal recessive pattern.

However, type 2B VWD results from a functionally abnormal von Willebrand factor molecule, whereas PT-VWD is caused by hyperresponsive platelets due to defects in the platelet GP1BA gene

Type 2A vWD has decreased platelet adhesion due to a selective deficiency of high molecular weight multimers and accounts for 20% to 25% of vWD.

Type 2A, which usually manifests as mild to
moderate mucocutaneous bleeding

Type 2B VWD is characterized by an abnormal von Willebrand factor protein with abnormally increased affinity to platelet GP1B that results in increased platelet aggregation, and increased proteolysis of von Willebrand factor subunits causing a decrease of large von Willebrand factor multimers.

In vWD type 2B, the abnormal von Willebrand factor spontaneously binds to GpIb in the absence of subendothelial contact.

Type 2B VWD is characterized by mild to moderate mucocutaneous bleeding that can include thrombocytopenia.

DDAVP trials may be contraindicated in patients with type IIB, because of thrombocytopenia and possible thrombotic complications.

Type 2M VWD is characterized by loss-of-function von Willebrand factor mutations that is characterized by decreased platelet adhesion without a deficiency in high molecular weight multimers. This functional mutation interfere with von Willebrand factor binding to platelets and/or subendothelium, causing a loss of function.

Type 2M vWD variant is characterized by a mild-moderate mucocutaneous bleeding that on can be severe.

Type 2N VWD creates a dysfunctional von Willebrand factor that has decreased binding affinity for factor VIII.

In vWD type IIN, the platelet-dependent functions of von Willebrand factor are normal but FVIII levels are low.

Type 2N VWD is associated with a Factor VIII deficiency characterized by Factor VIII levels that are disproportionally low when compared to the von Willebrand factor levels. Type 2N is different than the other type 2 variants of VWD, because is it autosomal recessive.

Type 2N VWD can manifest as excessive bleeding with surgery and in many respects is similar to mild hemophilia A.

In vWD type 3 disease there is almost complete absence of von Willebrand factor.

Type 3 VWD (<5% of VWD) manifests with severe mucocutaneous and musculoskeletal bleeding.

Type 3 vWD is inherited in a autosomal

recessive pattern.

Von Willebrand Type 3 is the most serious
form of VWD.

In pregnant patients with type 3 von Willebrand disease, the levels of von Willebrand factor will increase enough that there are usually no problems at the time of delivery. However postpartum GI bleeding may occur with NSAIDs.

Type 3 von Willebrand disease is associated with telangectasia, angiodysplasia of the intestinal wall, and mitral valve prolapse.

Patients with von Willebrand factor type 3 disease will also have low factor VIII levels and may develop arthropathies such as those seen commonly seen in hemophilia A.

Additional symptoms of type 3 vWD include nose bleeds, excessive bleeding after trauma, menorrhagia, hematuria, melena or hematochezia, large hematomas, and bleeding gums.

People with type 3 VWD usually are
diagnosed during their first year of life.

Acquired vWD is an uncommon disorder that is characterized by a late-onset bleeding diathesis in a patient with no prior bleeding history and a no family history of bleeding.

Acquired VWD is associated with decreased levels of factor VIII, von Willebrand factor antigen, and ristocetin cofactor activity.

Acquired vWD is usually associated with
another underlying disorder such as a
myeloproliferative disorder (with
thrombocytosis), hypothyroidism, benign or
malignant B-cell disorders, solid tumors
(Wilms tumor), cardiac or vascular defects.
Acquired vWD can be associated with drugs
such as ciprofloxacin and valproic acid.

This concludes Von Willebrand Disease: Fast Focus Study Guide

Search Amazon Kindle books to find other study guides written by

JT Thomas, MD

Internal Medicine Study Guide

Hematology Study Guide

Medical Oncology Study Guide

Cardiology Study Guide

Multiple Myeloma Study Guide

Differential Diagnosis Study Guide

Rheumatology Study Guide

Cancer Study Guide